HOW

TO LIVE

HEALTHY

BY EATING

HEALTHY

FOODS

TABLE OF CONTENTS

Disclaimer

INTRODUCTION

For some reason, eating healthfully is among the most difficult things a person can accomplish. There are several reasons why eating healthily is difficult, whether it be due to our lack of resources in many areas or the fact that junk food is readily available.

Yes, we can eat almost anything and it will keep us alive. We shall be able to function from one moment to the next and claim to be healthy. But is consuming processed meals and sugary beverages as a sole source of nutrition healthy? We should not assume that just because we are alive, we are healthy. And as we age, our unhealthy behaviors start to catch up with us more and more.

To avoid any potential problems in the future, it is crucial to establish good eating habits as early as possible in life. You don't want to discover one day that you've been suffering from a vitamin deficit for years and that it's led to consequences that are nearly impossible to treat. We all need to be more accountable for what we put into our bodies since failing to do so can be quite damaging.

A person can be the finest possible version of themselves, but if they don't even acknowledge that bad eating might derail them even in the present, they are eventually saying goodbye to the best future imaginable.However, anything can change. You will comprehend the significance of eating healthfully and how food affects our bodies and functions after reading this book.

It can be challenging to stay on track at times if you don't know why your body responds to food the way it does. But there are several ways you might start to comprehend the significance of consuming healthy meals and precisely how to start on a journey toward healthy eating. Let's stop wasting time now. We should start eating well right now!

Chapter:1 HOW WE THINK ABOUT FOOD

SYNOPSIS:

Even more important than an instructor, the most important item you need to keep your health and fitness program going is or a physician—is your own motivation. You must be tenacious. to examine the situation closely. Consequently, you are overweight and considering losing a couple pounds

If you don't take the necessary steps to have the proper diet and to adhere to your regular exercise schedule, no gym instructor from anywhere in the world will be able to help you. Even when you're ill and in pain No doctor will assist you with treatment if you aren't willing to adamant about adhering to the treatment plan, whether Taking the drug as directed or refraining from using some meals

YOUR MENTALITY:

So far, we have deviated drastically from our normal dietary patterns. Things won't go better unless we assess the situation and take action on our own.The most important factor is awareness. We must educate ourselves on which foods are healthy for us and which are not. We need to return to training and learn about the nutrients that

What your body actually craves and how much of it. Then we must create a nutrition plan ourselves and our family members so that we can eat well. We must cut. cut back on all things that are harmful, such as sweets, fats, and salt. the carbohydrates, which we don't actually desire - and include foods that could improve our health.

I realize that this does sound a bit overly preachy. However, that is the only break we have. We'll never get better as long as we keep eating Oreos. Still, there is hope. The fact that there are numerous foods available provides hope. that are just as delicious as those awful junk foods but we don't yet know about them. These are the foods that we don't know about yet, we likely don't care for them or as we don't know how to fix them, but a healthy cookbook may help you in understanding assorted interesting ways to healthy cooking. You can create some incredibly delectable healthy recipes even while maintaining the same type of diet you now follow. All of that is definitely feasible. You can significantly alter your dietary habits while maintaining or keeping your palate in mind at all times.The truth is that the weight loss industry has significantly contributed to the decline of the advanced human race. They must continue to sell their Jenny and Atkins' Because of Craigs, Zones, and Medi-fast, the You are never told how to interpret something in the media. hands.

Chapter 2:   Why Eat Healthy?

There are several reasons why eating healthily is vital. The majority of us are already aware of North America's growing obesity crisis. In general, this is especially true of the United States. The SAD diet is a term that describes the manner that many Americans eat.

SAD stands for standard American diet, and it refers to a diet low in vegetables, high in fat and sugar, and lacking in nutrition. Processed foods are definitely a part of the SAD diet. These are foods that are easily available and quick to consume and prepare but have long-lasting negative health effects.

Avoiding such processed meals and focusing instead on whole grains, fruits, vegetables, and meat that has not been treated with hormones or other chemicals that may ultimately find their way into your body and create problems is generally regarded as a good option if you want to prevent being obese. Unfortunately, there are many opportunities in North America for us to put off cooking meals.

We have so many items at our disposal, and purchasing poor quality food costs far less than purchasing high quality food. It may seem unusual that buying organic costs more than buying foods that may eventually lead to long-term health issues, but supply and demand dictate that this is the case. Additionally, due to their ease, processed foods are mass-produced and extremely profitable. Because of this, the obesity pandemic in North America is not entirely unexpected. On the list of businesses aiming to profit from people's lack of interest in cooking, nutrition is not at the top list of businesses looking to profit off consumers' indolence in the kitchen.

However, there are numerous benefits to eating well and compelling arguments against following the typical American diet and processed foods. For instance, you should absolutely check into the rest of this book to find strategies to modify your nutrition and start a healthy lifestyle if you do not want to be obese.

Healthy eating can also make you more vulnerable to illness. by eating unhealthy foods and by staying on a standard American diet that is full of fat and sugar. Diabetes is something that can be developed because of poor eating and can often times be treated with healthy eating.

In the end, type II diabetes is something that can be maintained and treated with healthy eating habits and is something that is started by unhealthy eating habits. Make an effort to make wise eating decisions if you want to stay away from these kinds of challenges and issues.

Poor eating can also lead to other ailments. Both chronic illnesses like high blood pressure and others are widespread. Because they didn't make proper food decisions earlier in life, osteoporosis is something that can afflict many people later in life. You can experience cardiac issues, high blood pressure, or poor bone health. All of which put a lot of stress on your body and can be extremely dangerous in the long run.

You should start making decisions now that will enable you to stay in their life for as long as possible if you want to demonstrate to your family that you care about them. Your poor health doesn't just affect you. It is something that also has an impact on those close to you. If they are watching you suffer because of poor choices that you have made, in a way, that is quite selfish. They are suffering too. Now, do your best to make the choices that will be the best not only for yourself, but for your family in the long run. This book will show you how.

Chapter 3: THE DANGERS OF OF FOLLOWING DIET TRENDS

Today's society is rife with diet trends, and almost all of them are associated with risks. Sadly, the majority of people who are eager to make money frequently ignore the long-term health effects of their products. Their primary interest is making money, and they are working to build something that will allow them to take advantage of the great need that many people have to lose weight quickly and easily.

If diet trends are something that pique your attention, there is something that you will have to accept.Unfortunately, there is no good technique to lose weight quickly and effortlessly without effort, a nutritious diet, or exercise. If you are overweight or in need of more mobility due to insufficient fitness, losing weight is a desirable objective.

Every one of us has occasionally required to begin making better lifestyle decisions, and we may accomplish this through eating well and engaging in regular physical activity rather than trusting businesses that wish to take advantage of us in order to profit.

Some of the current eating trends are extremely harmful and have severe long- and short-term health effects. Many of them rely on techniques that deprive Robert's body and ourselves of vital nutrients. even dehydrating us at times. These diet fads are abhorrent in every way. They are preying on those who desire health but lack the knowledge to get it. They prey on individuals, frequently women in particular, who are breaking under the weight of unattainable beauty standards and who are convinced that in order to be considered valuable, they need to appear a specific way.

That is wholly false. You have worth whether you are 100 or 700 pounds. However, eating healthily is one of the few effective methods you'll be able to jump-start your metabolism and provide your body the nutrition it needs to operate at its peak potential.

When you deprive your body of the vitamins and minerals it needs to survive and rely on a diet fad to educate you how to slim down and feel good when all they actually want is your cash, you will find yourself more behind than when you started. The unpleasant reality is that many diet fads send the body into famine mode and can damage your metabolism, making you acquire weight more quickly in the future. Don't let the advertising that claim to help you lose weight quickly and easily trick you. easy method All of that will be expensive. Additionally, there are health fads out there, like the HCG diet, that can seriously mess with your body and hormones.

Diet trends are hilarious in that they frequently lead to unhealthy and challenging methods of weight maintenance, which will make it more difficult for you to lose weight in the future. Do not believe a drug you see advertised on television if you want to lose weight. Replace unhealthy processed and sugary foods with whole-grain alternatives and organic fruits and vegetables to avoid introducing chemicals into your body that will make it more difficult for you to lose weight and ultimately disrupt your body chemistry

Being able to drop pounds rapidly without having to give up the unhealthy eating habits you have accumulated over the years may seem alluring, but it is unhealthy. If you are not careful about the manner you attempt to reduce weight, you are harming yourself and setting up your body for future health issues. Be sure to take all reasonable steps to make decisions that you would want others to make for themselves..

Before you succumb to the TV snake oil salesman, do some homework. Look into these issues because you deserve to do things correctly and because you don't want your future to be muddled by the negative repercussions of a sales pitch that just cares about your wallet and not your wellbeing.

CHAPTER 4: FOLLOWING THE FOOD PYRAMID

Most of us have likely seen the food pyramid. Growing up, the meals pyramid was once often used as a guideline for us to supply us with an thought of how an awful lot meals and what form of food we ought to eat each and every day in order to preserve a healthy lifestyle.

Of course, there is usually evidence to country that the meals pyramid is flexible, but overall, if you are in a position to take a look at the food pyramid you will have a regular idea of what is ideal in a healthful and nutritious diet. While this would possibly also moreover additionally now and as soon as greater be controversial, it is nevertheless fantastic to have a quintessential food. Possibly one that you create yourself. A lot of human beings will say that it is no longer viewed the most healthy problem to do to consume as many grains as the foods pyramid may also moreover moreover have suggested.

In fact, with current outbreaks of celiac disease, a lot of human beings are touting a no grain lifestyle as the most healthful choice. Rather than relying on the meals pyramid for your easy guiding precept of what is healthful to eat, try to take into consideration your ownnon-public experiences with food and go from there. Some humans are healthier with a lot of grains, and some are not. Use your judgment here to the pleasant of your capability so that you will be able to take steps in the proper path for your health.

The wellknown meals pyramid recommends as follows:

• Rice, cereal, pasta, and bread, can be as many as eleven servings per day.

• For veggies and fruits, you have to have between three and 5 servings.

• As a ways as their eggs, you can have two or three servings each day, supplied you are now not allergic or lactose intolerant.

• When it comes to meet and beans, and other things like nuts and fish or poultry, it is encouraged that you have two or three servings each and every day.

• Unsurprisingly, things such as sugar and fat and oil are the very tip of the. Because you have to now not have any of these matters in excess. Rather, use them only as indispensable in order to assurance your healthiest feasible lifestyle.

Again, this is only referencing the general food pyramid. Depending on your personal singular wishes and dietary functions, you may need to modify this chart for yourself. But if you do not have any unique requirements, this is the wellknown for the food

pyramid that can be utilized to your best possible gain in growing a healthier lifestyle.

Chapter 5: THE HEALTH BENEFITS OF EATING FRUITS AND VEGETABLES

FRUITS

It is an unlucky but common understanding that human beings who follow the general American diet do not eat ample fruit. What fruit they do eat is normally discovered in cans or saturated with sugar. The added sugar and fruit is truely something that takes away any fitness advantages that consuming fruit in its natural kingdom can furnish the body.

There can be some complications to eating too a great deal fruit, specially if you have diabetes. Fruit is high in natural sugars, and when it is juiced, you get a lot of sugar without a lot of fiber, which can grant the body with an excess.

The fiber current inside fruit is one of the things that makes it the healthiest, and helps the physique to lower heart disorder and keep away from constipation. Not solely that, but fiber rich meals like fruit and vegetables are very advisable for weight administration due to the fact it helps you to feel full with fewer calories. Not only that, but fruit is high in many vitamins and minerals, specially citrus fruits when it comes to vitamin C

Vitamin C is a powerhouse when it comes to supporting the body to heal, and if you want some thing that will help you to keep your enamel and gums healthy, vitamin C wealthy fruits will truly do the trick.

Another issue that fruit can help the body obtain is stroke prevention and kidney stone prevention. Fruits are very useful in assisting the body and preventing and hostilities disorders such as pores and skin conditions and heart problems. Fruit can be one of the most wholesome approaches to assist you to get a raise of power and get rid of sugar cravings that you may have when you are trying to cut unhealthy ingredients out of your diet.

As long as you aren't overdoing it with your fruits, such as throwing a bunch of them in the blender and sooner or later ingesting a ridiculous quantity of sugar, then you can have a healthy snack that satisfies your candy tooth if you are willing to make use of the fantastic strength of fruit.

If you are involved in the advantages that food can have to your health, both fruits and vegetables have a herbal tendency to help your skin glow and appear a ways more hydrated and nourished. Fruits and veggies are excessive in antioxidants and vitamins and minerals that supply your body with the hydration essential in preserving your pores and skin and look healthy. It can help your hair to grow softer and more healthy, as nicely as retaining the youthful appear of your skin. Fruit can even help you

to end pimples in its tracks by way of preserving your body free of waste products that come out thru your pores and hydrating your skin. Fruit is outstanding for supporting the physique to stay hydrated because of its excessive water content, and you will shortly commence to see the advantages and that aspect.

VEGETABLES

Vegetables are one of the most under-sung meals in existence, specifically when it comes to the standard American diet. Most humans don't realize just how necessary it is to furnish the physique with the nutritional vitamins and minerals that greens and veggies on my own can provide. Sometimes, human beings will appear into veggies as a way of enhancing their beauty, however when it comes to improving their health, they come to be truly disinterested.

However, now that you are here and studying this book, it is secure to assume that you are willing and capable to take into consideration why it is important to consume vegetables. Here are some of the quality motives to provide your self with veggies daily as a part of your diet.

First of all, the physique wishes fiber in order to get rid of excess waste. Without a way to discover the waste collectively and eliminated, it stays caught in the physique and can make contributions to weight reap and other doable complications.

Fiber is extraordinarily necessary for other reasons as well. It can assist you to forestall your blood cholesterol from elevating and can even prevent heart disease, or at least decrease the probabilities of struggling from it.

Folic acid is additionally current in vegetables, and when you are presenting your physique with this substance, it can generate the manufacturing of your crimson blood cells. This can be very vital in assisting you to prevent anemia from occurring, and can be very really useful to women in particular, who have a tendency to need this substance at some point of pregnancy and menstruation.

Vegetables are also naturally excessive in many vitamins, such as a and C, which are beneficial in warfare infection and maintaining the physique healthy. It can assist you to speed up the recovery manner and to soak up iron, which is every other way of helping to combat and prevent anemia from occurring. Vitamins are high in potassium and this is very useful because it prevents the physique from succumbing to high blood pressure.

Vegetables have been verified to reduce the danger of strokes and different heart associated complications. They can stop kidney stones from creating and forestall the disintegration of bone matter. Filling yourself up on vegetables is a properly way to help you to manipulate kind II diabetes and obesity.

Not solely that, but it can assist you to continue to be sturdy in a combat against most cancers and in cancer prevention. Perhaps one of the mostredeeming qualities about ingesting vegetables is the truth that they are very low in fats and are sincerely now not calorie dense.

This potential that you can consume as many vegetables as you favor to without having to worry too a whole lot about gaining weight. Snacking on vegetables is a super way to help you to minimize starvation cravings and to stay targeted on a healthful lifestyle.

There are so many extremely good matters about vegetables. It is shocking that they are so uncommon to come via in the general American diet. One of the first-class ways that you can help yourself in heading off high fats and high sugar and high salt processed foods is in taking walks round the outdoor of your grocery save first.

Go alongside the sparkling produce part so that you are making conscious options in imparting your body with healthful sparkling vegetable preferences as a substitute than skipping to the end and cheating via shopping for pastas and other processed ingredients that are low in in reality nutritious vegetable content.

Healthy ingesting begins with making the alternatives to nourish your body, and there are few things extra nourishing than vegetables.

We can regularly lose our taste for healthful meals due to the fact of unhealthy and terrible consuming habits early in life, or even self-imposed later in life, but it is easy to get lower back on track. Make time in your lifestyles for vegetables. They may also take a little bit longer to prepare, however the benefits are well worth it.

Top Fruits and Vegetables That Improve Athletic Performance

Beets

Beets are a long way and away amongst the very most vital greens for

building muscle and for athletes of all kinds. That's because beets are amongst the most superb meals in the world when it comes to elevating nitric oxide. Nitric oxide is a natural 'vasodilator'. This ability that it can motive the blood vessels (veins and arteries) to dilate (widen) thereby encouraging the glide of oxygen and nutrients round the body.

The result is that the muscle groups get more oxygen and power in the course of training and more nutrients for enhancing recovery. This can assist you elevate for extra reps, run further distances and recover at a quicker rate.

Potatoes

Carbohydrates are frequently made out to be the bad guys but in reality they are very important for constructing muscle and for physical training in general. Potatoes are a good desire of carbohydrate because they're additionally excessive in fiber, excessive in vitamin C (which enhances recovery) and low in calories. Consume after a exercising and the energy will go straight to the muscle tissues instead than the waist. This is important seeing as diet D is considered to be a master hormone regulator, and is responsible for encouraging the production of testosterone in particular – one of the predominant anabolic hormones for constructing muscle and burning

fat.

What's more, is that diet D has these days been shown to be a good deal more effective than even vitamin C when it comes to assisting the immune device and preventing colds and flus. As any athlete knows, a bloodless can be adequate to complete derail and athletes training plan, which in turn can be the distinction between victory and failure!

Carrots

Carrots are commonly healthy and a magnificent supply of diet A, C and K. What's really exciting about them even though is the lutein, which may help to make bigger energy levels and beautify the efficiency of your very mitochondria! Your mitochondria are the energy factories of your cells which convert glucose into ATP (glucose being the sugar that comes from carbs, and ATP being the usable structure of strength in your body). This in short means that with carrots and other sources of lutein, you can simply run faster and that you'll definitely burn more energy even when you're resting! In one study, rats have been given lutein (which wishes a supply of fats to soak up such as milk) and it used to be located that they started running lengthy distances voluntarily in their wheel, burning a whole lot more fats as they did.

Apples

Apples are prosperous in diet C, which is some other indispensable nutrition for improving the immune system and helping athletes teach longer and harder except fail.

Vitamin C additionally helps to encourage the restore of muscle tissue, will increase serotonin to aid with mental recovery, and even will increase the manufacturing of both testosterone and nitric oxide when paired with zinc.

Chapter 6: The Dangers in The Excessive Intake of Processed Foods

It does no longer come as a shock to all people that processed ingredients are dangerous. What does come as a surprise on the other hand is that they are nonetheless allowed out on the shelves, no matter the havoc that they wreak on our bodies and minds. Eating unhealthy food isn't just a private choice to some people.

Sometimes, due to the fact of the way the economic system works, humans in poverty are forced to flip to processed ingredients due to the fact they are a cheap and convenient way to feed massive families on a low budget.

The hard thing about that is that these meals in the end cause medical troubles down the line that cost even greater cash than it would take to feed a large family healthy, sustainable options. Ultimately, it seems that human beings with little money are suffering both way.

Even if you don't have to feed a household on a budget, processed ingredients are truly unhealthy. Part of what makes them so addicting is their high fat and sugar content.

They are often boxed foods that encompass pastas and an super quantity of sugar. Excessive sugar is hazardous in general, however specifically to people who are prone to growing type II diabetes. If you eat sugar and excessive amounts, you are ultimately going to overload your body and not solely will you become obese, extra than likely, but you also enhance fitness issues.

Sugar can help velocity along the manner of diabetes because of the fact that it reasons insulin resistance to appear which in the end makes it difficult, if not impossible, to manipulate your blood sugar levels.

If you consume ingredients like this excessively, such as for each and every meal, or at least each and every day, there is bound to be a poor consequence. Consuming that excessive amount of fat and sugar on a consistent foundation can lead to no longer solely diabetes and obesity, which are often known, however also coronary heart disease and even cancer. This is enormously dangerous, and if possible, processed ingredients should be avoided at all costs.

Another threat of ingesting processed foods is that now not only are they addicting, however they are relatively artificial. Most of the substances in these ingredients are now not nourishing the body. Rather, they are main us to experience full whilst depriving our bodies of the imperative nutrients that are required in healthful functioning.

When we are ingesting a food regimen that is bland and not nourishing, we are sooner or later permitting ourselves to be dumbed down. We are not questioning properly, we are now not moving properly, and we are not functioning at her very best viable potential. All of these things are highly negative and can lead to poor coordination and even depression.

On some level, we all recognize that processed meals are now not as wholesome as the sorts of ingredients we should be consuming on a everyday basis. Our bodies recognize it, even if our minds are now not aware. And we go through for it. We have stress about it.

When we indulge in unhealthy foods, whether or not we are addicted to them or not, our bodies recognize it. And, whether it's a unconscious occurrence or not, we frequently punish ourselves. We recognize that we are doing some thing wrong. We experience upset about it and dissatisfied, even if we are processing it in the moment.

Processed ingredients are also excessive in synthetic colorings that have been established to be fairly carcinogenic. When we are consuming meals that have fixed coloring in it, we are actually swallowing dye. Would you want to eat hair dye? Not really. But these kinds of chemicals are what are used in your food. They remain in your physique and do now not come out. They dye your organs on the inside. They are distinctly unsafe and can lead to cancer.

There also full of preservatives. Processed meals stays on the shelf for a very long time. Longer than is healthy and normal. Any

typical bottle of milk would now not closing for months on give up at a time. It would curdle and spoil. The identical as with cheeses, and the identical as with other foods that you discover on the shelves that have lengthy shelf lives.

Shelf lives are important for agencies to establish because they are able to make greater money if their food is able to remain on the shelf longer. They will do anything it takes, whether or not it is healthier now not to the human body, to ensure that they are making the most money possible.

Preservatives regularly encompass unhealthy and unnatural chemicals and immoderate amounts of salt. Neither of which are exact for the physique at all. Processed ingredients can lead to troubles with the heart, and hypertension, due to the fact of the immoderate amount of salt existing in these foods. High blood stress is a frequent occurrence among human beings who continue to exist off of processed foods, and weight problems and heart attacks are some of the wide variety one killer's in North America.

This has truely the entirety to do with the popular American diet. The sad phase about it is that even if you recognize it is unhealthy, the chemical substances and excessive sugar and fat content make these processed ingredients extraordinarily addicting.

The body begins to crave them, and it can be nearly as hazardous as a drug addiction. When you are addicted to a food that is neither nourishing nor healthy, it can have long-term penalties on your fitness and development.

Another way that processed ingredients contribute to weight problems is due to the fact we digest them far too shortly in contrast to meals that are prosperous in healthy dietary fiber. If we are digesting these foods shortly and they are now not filling us up due to the fact we are now not receiving the fiber that affords us with the full feeling, we are not even burning the equal quantity of power as we would to digest healthy foods.

This capacity that we consume extra and digest less, leading to quickly and fast weight gain. The energy current in your physique are tons greater when you are on a weight-reduction plan of processed foods. You burn some distance extra calories when you are consuming healthy, total ingredients that are rich in dietary fibers.

Unfortunately, this means that people who live and subsist on a food regimen of processed meals are in the end going to acquire weight whether they desire to or not. And they will now not grant you with the same amount of power because they are not nourishing. They are probable to leave you worn-out and sluggish, and feeling some distance too full due to the fact you devour a lot more of these unhealthy, sugar crammed ingredients barring feeling content or satiated.

Processed meals is not metabolized proper in our bodies. They are shortly became to fat. Not solely that, but they are excessive in fat. They are frequently full of hidden fats and sugars

Chapter 7: How Food can become Medicine

The same way that now not eating wholesome can make you sick, ingesting wholesome foods can frequently instances remedy you of sickness and grant you with relief when you are suffering.

It can additionally act as a preventative measure to take against illness. In fact, there is an entire approach of healing round India for lots of years referred to as Aryuveda.

This historical recuperation fashion is utilized in order to treat any sickness certainly by altering your diet. Food is actually the medicinal drug that has helped to preserve the humans of India alive for centuries. And it can nevertheless be applicable today.

In fact, many treatments are simply healthful ingredients that have anti-inflammatory homes and the capacity to nourish your body from the inner out. Everything from contamination to most cancers has been acknowledged to be impacted by means of healthful consuming choices.

And with this historic recovery art, that has by no means been greater apparent. Of route a lot of present day technology will frown upon these techniques due to the fact they have not been scientifically investigated, but a lot of it has been tried and authentic for hundreds of years and will proceed to have an impact on the body.

Whether you trust in the ancient recovery artwork or not, the truth stays that meals can finally determine whether or no longer you are inclined to illness. If you eat well, your physique will be better and it will be capable to battle off illness and contamination a ways less difficult than it would if you locate yourself malnourished on popular American diet.

Without the acceptable nutritional vitamins and minerals in your body, it can be nearly impossible to combat off the terrible consequences of illness. Sometimes, it can even purpose illness. If you are ingesting unhealthy unprocessed foods, certain sorts of these ingredients can virtually lead to illnesses and make you more inclined to certain kinds of cancer as well.

Although most cancers is nevertheless being researched and has no longer wholly been understood through the scientific community well adequate to absolutely therapy it, there are many cases of people who were in a position to live lengthy and healthy lives truely by using altering the way they need. Healthy consuming can help in decreasing the signs and symptoms of many challenging and impossible to remedy diseases, such as more than one sclerosis.

As long as you are making sure that everything that you put into your physique is nourishing and is presenting your organs and cells with all of the fuel and sources that they need in order to keep your body strong, they will proceed to do that. And they will do it to the exceptional of their ability.

However, if you are actively sabotaging your body, they will no longer be able to put up the equal fight as they would if they had been receiving ample nutrition. That is why it is so important for you to take heed of the way you are nourishing your body. If you are now not making active and conscientious selections about the food that you eat, you could be setting your self up for failure in ways that you may additionally live to regret.

Chapter: 8 PUTTING IT ALL TOGETHER WITH MEAL PLANNING/ FORMULATION

Meal planning can be one of the single most vital aspects of developing a healthful lifestyle. When we are unable to visualize the future of our eating, it can be very easy to succumb to the temptations of unhealthy ingredients that we have turn out to be addicted to. Especially if it is our habit to devour them instead than eating the ingredients that will nourish us.

Meal planning is pretty an endeavor. It can be really intimidating, specially to any individual who suffers with organization. If you locate yourself having a hard time with meal planning, don't fret. There are many methods that you can commence to delve into meal planning that are fun and easy, whether you war with creativity in the kitchen or not.

There are many meal planning kits that you can buy. Many of them have the alternative of ordering boxes full of sparkling meals to prepare dinner with and consist of recipes that you can use. This can be very helpful if you are not used to cooking, which is often the case.

Especially when poor eating habits and a busy work agenda make it seem tough to carve out the time indispensable in order to make full, nourishing meals. The first step in meal planning is research. If you are going to get yourself healthy, you have to look at your options.

Researching recipes is the satisfactory first area to start. Accumulating a binder full of healthy meals that you choose to attempt out can be each fun and educational. It will open your mind to numerous meals possibilities you can also have otherwise scoffed at as too challenging for you to prepare, or possibly instruct you things you had in no way recognized before.

Recipes can be very mind-opening. Especially when you are

interested in making new discoveries. Cooking can be a hard addiction to get into, however as soon as you commence to grasp it, you will be amazed by just how a whole lot freedom you can locate in putting a meal collectively for your self that is each health-conscious and delicious!

Look at recipe books and magazines and get an accumulation of recipes that you prefer to try. Start with the things that look the most scrumptious and nourishing, and if you are a novice in the kitchen, you may additionally also favor to seem to the things that appear the most simple.

Next, you ought to maintain your recipes organized in a simple way that is convenient to navigate. If you discover yourself overwhelmed by way of a lack of organization, it will make meal planning that tons extra difficult.

When you are commencing a new habit, you prefer to make positive that you are doing the entirety as truely as possible. Too tons alternate at once can be stressful on your system, and you need to always attempt to put in force small, handy modifications till they have turn out to be a new habit.

Make sure that they are easily accessible, so that when you desire to begin getting ready your meal you can do so easily. If you are using a binder, you may additionally favor to think about laminating the pages or the use of plastic sleeves, so that if you are using it in the kitchen, they are now not affected via water or other meals contamination.

When you organize your recipes, it would help to put them in order of breakfast meals, lunch meals, dinner meals, and snacks. This will assist you to reference the proper recipes more without problems as soon as you commence to start cooking. If you like, you ought to even prepare your binder by way of day of the week, and have your ingredients deliberate out for each and every day and printed out in the binder that way.

There are many methods you should organize your recipes. Do what appears to make the most experience to you intuitively. Don't pressure yourself to adhere to a type of agency that doesn't work for you. Instead, make sure that you are doing what works fantastic for you in your personal life.

Make positive that you are taking the time to oftentimes seek out new recipes that stand out to you to hold your creative juices flowing and your kitchen exciting. There are many sorts of recipes you can try, and the extra you attempt, the extra interesting going on a experience of healthful eating can be!

Next, you discover software program such as Excel on Microsoft Office that will help you to prepare your meal planning. On Excel you will find a plethora of templates you can choose from to assist your self diagram out your meals through the day, time, and week. This can be a vastly valuable resource!

If you would select no longer to use excel, there are additionally apps you ought to download on your smartphone, tablet or some other machine to assist you to make use of your time and sources better.

You can even go the old normal route and purchase a notebook that is in particular designed toward planning meals. This is an vital step in making sure your foods are organized and effortlessly accessible.

Having a meal format is extremely helpful when it comes to embarking upon a ride of healthful eating. Creating precise habits takes time and patience, and it is inevitable that you will slip somewhere alongside the way.

But that doesn't imply that you have to remain caught on the ground! Actually, it just capability that you are going to have to get returned up and keep trying, because giving up is far less difficult than sticking to your plans.

One issue that can truely assist when it comes to meal planning is sticking with the theme. For example, a lot of human beings have precise issues like taco Tuesday or another day that is assigned for a unique kind of meal. If you assume that would assist you to remain on track, feel free to imitate that kind of meal planning. It is executed for a reason, because it works and it helps to maintain things simple and streamlined.

It can be very stressful to locate yourself stuck doing a lot of planning and education every single week or month, so if you choose to preserve matters easy, that can be a proper way to do it. You may want to have a theme for biweekly meals, such as taco Tuesday one night time and maybe rice and veggies Tuesday the next and alternate between them. There is no wrong way to design your meals. What you have to make sure you do is to have a look at comply with through.

Without follow-through, the entirety else will become redundant and difficult. Something that can surely help you to prevail at meal planning is accountability. If you let anyone who is aware of you and cares about you know that you are attempting to plan your meals, ask them if they would be willing to help you to stick to your routine.

They can assist you with the aid of asking questions about how things are going and whether or not or now not you are staying on track. They might also additionally select to motivate you and cheer you on via your endeavors.

Conclusion

Healthy eating is some thing that can be very challenging to begin doing, in particular if you were not able to improve healthful consuming habits from a younger age. However, it is not impossible to become a more health conscious and proactive person.

Fortunately, every single day that we wake up living and respiratory is a day that we can start to higher ourselves and move forward in our lives.

Becoming the fantastic model of ourselves can seem intimidating at first, but as soon as you start to realise that each and every desire you make has an have an effect on on your life, whether superb or negative, then it will become a lot easier to see the path of our actions before they come again to haunt us. Poor ingesting habits are certainly selections that will come again to hang-out us.

If we are now not careful, we will begin to improve fitness issues later in lifestyles because we had been now not conscientious of what we put into our bodies when we were younger. Healthy consuming and exercise is the solely way to create a wholesome and blissful physique and mind.

We end up stir loopy and stressed when we remain stuck in our properties all day consuming nothing however sugar and fats laden processed ingredients and sitting round looking at TV except exercising. The standard American eating regimen is dangerous, and it is costing human beings their lives. Don't let your self come to be one of these people.

Instead, make the selections that you need to make in order to actually higher your self and come to be the high-quality model of your self possible. Make picks that will make your family proud and will supply them with your presence in their lives for years to come.

With all that said, right here is your blueprint to enhance your health and happiness hugely by getting more fruits and vegetables:

Start your day with a smoothie, but don't have more than one fruit smoothie Don't purpose to get just 5-7 fruits and veggies in your diet. Get as many as you can in order to get a varied mix.

 Use a supplement as a "back up." This is additionally mainly useful when seeking out greater dim and rare nutrients.

But make positive that you read the instructions and do your very own research. You may also wish to think about timing and adding a source of fat to aid absorption.

 Use techniques to make it as handy as viable to get more fruits and vegetables in your diet. Avoid processed meals and "empty calories" – exchange matters like chips and chocolate bars with salads and carrot sticks

Maintain this software for 30 days. You should discover you note you have more energy, drive, and better health. Use this new energy to improve your lifestyle in other ways!

SUMMARY

It can be challenging to stay on track at times if you don't know why your body responds to food the way it does. But there are several ways you might start to comprehend the significance of consuming healthy meals and precisely how to start on a journey toward healthy eating.